Welcome!

Thank you for picking up this book and taking the first step toward fueling your fitness goals with delicious, high-protein meals. Whether you're just starting your fitness journey or looking to elevate your meal prep game, this book is here to make high-protein eating simple, flavorful, and effective. Each recipe is crafted to help you build muscle, boost energy, and keep you feeling strong inside and outside the gym. Let this book be your guide and companion on the path to a healthier, stronger you.

A Note of Gratitude

This book wouldn't have been possible without the love, encouragement, and support of our incredible friends and family. To each of you who has cheered us on, believed in us, and reminded us of our potential, we are endlessly grateful. Your kindness and faith in us are what keep us going. We love you all more than words can express—thank you for being our foundation and our inspiration.

Jai Lee

ByJaiLee.com

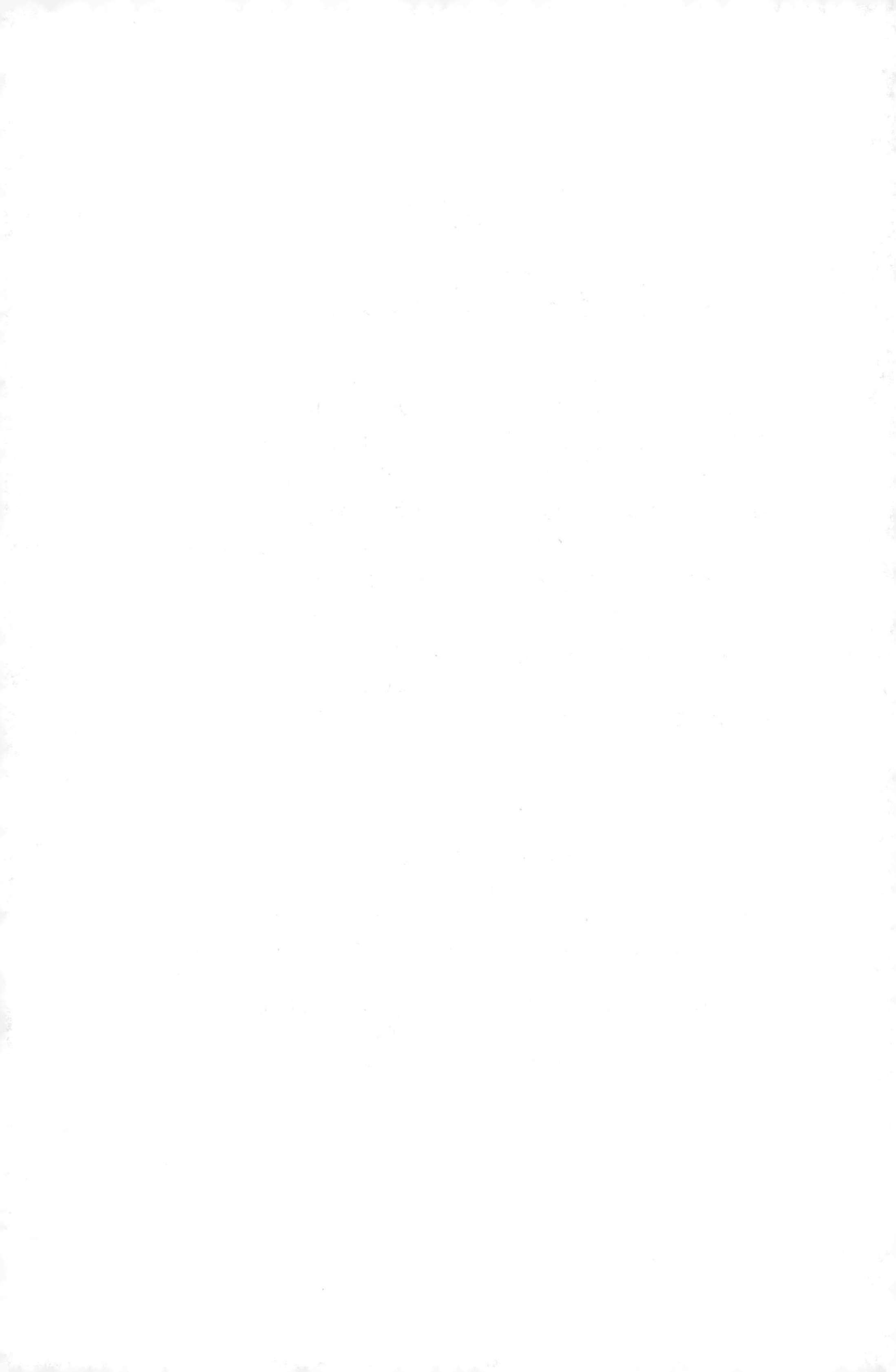

TABLE OF CONTENTS

<u>Food Disclaimer</u>

The recipes provided in this book are for informational purposes only and are intended to offer a general guide to cooking. While we strive to ensure all recipes are accurate and safe, we cannot guarantee that the instructions will suit every individual's needs or circumstances; so feel free to tweak them to your liking.

<u>Important Considerations:</u>

1. Allergies and Dietary Restrictions:
• Always check the ingredients for potential allergens before preparing any recipe. If you have specific dietary restrictions or allergies, substitute ingredients accordingly.
2. Food Safety:
• Follow standard food safety practices. Ensure all meats are cooked to the appropriate temperatures, and all fruits and vegetables are washed thoroughly before use.
• Avoid cross-contamination by using separate utensils and cutting boards for raw and cooked foods. Also, be sure to wash your hands and maintain a clean working area.
3. Nutritional Information:
• Nutritional values provided are estimates and can vary based on quantity and quality. For precise dietary advice, consult a registered dietitian or nutritionist.
4. Health Concerns:
• Consult with your healthcare provider before making significant changes to your diet, especially if you have any underlying health conditions.

The authors and publishers of this book are not responsible for any adverse reactions, effects, or health issues resulting from the use of recipes or ingredients mentioned in this book. Use these recipes at your own risk and discretion.

Elevate Your Goals

Get Fit, Stay Inspired, Stay Strong

Your body is your most valuable asset, and exercise is one of the greatest ways to honor and care for it. Regular movement isn't just about building muscle or losing weight—it transforms your life from the inside out.

Exercise boosts your energy, strengthens resilience, enhances your mood, and improves longevity by supporting heart health and overall vitality. It teaches discipline, builds confidence, and reveals strength you never knew you had.

It's not about perfection—it's about showing up for yourself. Every effort is a step toward a healthier, happier, and stronger you. Let this book guide and inspire you on your journey. You've got this!

START HERE

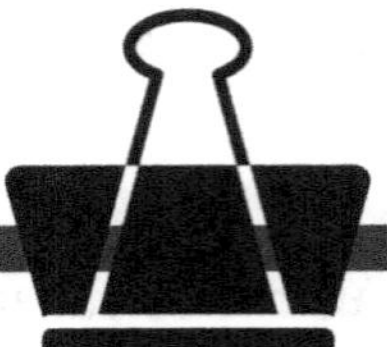

What's your favorite high-protein meal?

____

____

How do you plan your meals to support your fitness goals?

____

____

What's your go-to pre- or post-workout snack?

____

____

How do you balance nutrition with your workout routine?

____

____

What fitness goal motivates you to keep going?

____

____

BREAKFAST

Breakfast is the fuel your body needs to start the day strong. A high-protein breakfast boosts energy, enhances focus, supports muscle recovery, and stabilizes blood sugar levels, setting you up for a more productive and balanced day.

TURKEY & EGG BREAKFAST BURRITO

BELIEVE IN YOURSELF!

1
SERVING

33g
PROTEIN

INGREDIENTS	NOTES
• 3 large eggs **(18g protein)** • 2oz lean turkey sausage **(12g protein)** • 1 whole-grain tortilla **(3g protein)** • Season to taste	Optional: For extra flavor, you can add 1/4 cup shredded cheese **(7g protein)**, salsa, or hot sauce. Refrigerator Option: Refrigerate in an airtight container for up to 2-3 days. Freeze Option: Wrap tight with foil or plastic wrap. Store up to 1-2 months.

DIRECTIONS

1. Prepare the Sausage:
• Heat a non-stick skillet over medium heat.
• Add the turkey sausage and cook for 4-5 minutes, breaking it into small crumbles with a spatula, until fully cooked and browned. Remove from the pan and set aside.

2. Cook the Eggs:
• In a small bowl, whisk the eggs until smooth.
• Pour the eggs into the same skillet and cook over medium heat, stirring occasionally, until scrambled and fully cooked.

3. Assemble the Burrito:
• Lay the whole-grain tortilla flat on a plate.
• Add the scrambled eggs and cooked sausage to the center of the tortilla.

4. Wrap the Burrito:
  Fold in the sides of the tortilla and roll it tightly into a burrito shape.

EGG AND VEGGIE SCRAMBLE

KEEP PUSHING FORWARD!

1 SERVING

32g PROTEIN

INGREDIENTS	NOTES
• 4 large eggs **(24g protein)** • 1/2 cup cooked spinach **(2g protein)** • 1 oz feta cheese **(4g protein)** • 1/4 cup diced bell peppers **(0.5g protein)** • 1/4 cup diced zucchini **(0.5g protein)** • 1/4 cup chopped mushrooms **(1g protein)** • Season to taste	Optional: 1 slice whole-grain toast **(3g protein)**. Refrigerator Option: Refrigerate leftovers for up to 3 days. Freeze Option: Store in an airtight container for up to 1 month.

DIRECTIONS

1. Prepare the Vegetables:
• Heat a non-stick skillet over medium heat. Add olive oil if needed.
• Sauté the bell peppers, zucchini, and mushrooms for 3-4 minutes, or until tender.

2. Cook the Spinach:
  Add the cooked spinach to the skillet with the other vegetables and stir for 1-2 minutes until heated through.

3. Scramble the Eggs:
• In a bowl, whisk the eggs until smooth.
• Push the vegetables to one side of the skillet, then pour the eggs into the other side.
• Stir gently to scramble the eggs, gradually mixing in the vegetables as they cook.

4. Add Feta Cheese:
  Once the eggs are almost set, sprinkle the feta cheese over the scramble. Stir gently until combined.

PEANUT BUTTER PROTEIN SMOOTHIE

STRENGTH STARTS TODAY!

1 SERVING

32g PROTEIN

INGREDIENTS	NOTES
<ul><li>1 scoop whey protein powder **(20g protein)**</li><li>1 cup unsweetened almond milk **(1g protein)**</li><li>1 tbsp peanut butter **(4g protein)**</li><li>1/4 cup plain Greek yogurt **(5g protein)**</li><li>1/2 frozen banana **(0.5g protein)**</li><li>1 tbsp chia seeds **(2g protein)**</li><li>Ice cubes (optional, for texture)</li></ul>	Spice Options: Nutmeg, cinnamon, ginger, pumpkin spice. Refrigerator Option: Refrigerate prepared smoothies for up to 24 hours. Freeze Option: Freeze the ingredients (without almond milk and ice) in a bag and blend them when ready.

DIRECTIONS

1. Prepare Ingredients:
Gather all ingredients and make sure the banana is frozen for a creamier texture.

2. Blend:
Add the whey protein powder, almond milk, peanut butter, Greek yogurt, frozen banana, chia seeds, and ice cubes (if using) to a blender.

3. Blend Smooth:
Blend on high speed for 30-60 seconds, or until smooth and creamy.

4. Serve:
Pour into a glass and serve immediately.

PROTEIN PANCAKES
WITH BLUEBERRIES

FOCUS ON GROWTH! | **1** SERVING | **35g** PROTEIN

INGREDIENTS

- 1 scoop whey protein powder **(20g protein)**
- 1/4 cup rolled oats (**3g protein**)
- 1 large egg + 2 egg whites **(12g protein)**
- 1/4 cup unsweetened almond milk
- 1/4 cup fresh or frozen blueberries
- 1/2 tsp baking powder
- Season to taste

NOTES

Optional Toppings (to boost flavor and protein):
- 1/4 cup plain Greek yogurt **(5g protein)**
- 1 tbsp almond butter or peanut butter **(4g protein)**
- 1/2 tsp vanilla extract

Refrigerator Option: Store for up to 3 days.

Freeze Option: Stack pancakes with parchment paper in between and wrap them in foil or plastic wrap for up to 1 month.

DIRECTIONS

1. Prepare the Batter:
• Blend the protein powder, oats, egg, egg whites, almond milk, baking powder, and vanilla extract (if using) in a blender until smooth.
• Gently fold in the blueberries by hand after blending.

2. Cook the Pancakes:
• Heat a non-stick skillet or griddle over medium heat and lightly coat with cooking spray or oil.
• Pour 1/4 cup of batter onto the skillet for each pancake.
• Cook for 2-3 minutes or until bubbles form on the surface, then flip and cook the other side for 1-2 minutes until golden brown.

3. Serve:
  Stack the pancakes on a plate and top with additional blueberries, Greek yogurt, or nut butter for added flavor and protein.

GREEK YOGURT PARFAIT W/ PROTEIN GRANOLA

DISCIPLINE FUELS SUCCESS! | **1** SERVING | **33g** PROTEIN

INGREDIENTS	NOTES
<ul><li>1 cup non-fat Greek yogurt **(20g protein)**</li><li>1/4 cup high-protein granola **(10g protein)**</li><li>1/2 cup mixed berries (e.g., blueberries, strawberries</li><li>1 tsp honey or maple syrup for sweetness</li><li>1 tbsp chopped nuts or seeds, such as almonds or chia seeds **(2-3g protein)**</li></ul>	Optional:<ul><li>2 tbsp chia seeds **(5g protein)**</li><li>3 tbsp hemp seeds **(10g protein)**</li><li>Cinnamon, nutmeg</li></ul>Refrigerator Option: Store the yogurt and granola in the refrigerator separately for 1-2 days. Assemble the parfait before eating. Do not freeze.

DIRECTIONS

1. Prepare Ingredients:
• Wash the berries and pat them dry.
• Gather the yogurt, granola, and toppings for layering.

2. Layer the Parfait:
• In a mason jar or bowl, spoon half of the Greek yogurt as the first layer.
• Add a layer of berries, followed by a layer of protein granola.
• Repeat with the remaining yogurt, berries, and granola to create a beautiful layered effect.

3. Add Final Touches:
• Drizzle honey or maple syrup on top if you want a touch of sweetness.
• Sprinkle chopped nuts or seeds for added crunch and protein, if desired.

4. Serve:
 Serve immediately with a spoon, or refrigerate for up to 1 hour if you prefer it chilled.

HIGH-PROTEIN OVERNIGHT OATS

BREAK YOUR LIMITS! | **1** SERVING | **42g** PROTEIN

INGREDIENTS	NOTES
<ul><li>½ cup rolled oats **(5g protein)**</li><li>½ cup nonfat Greek yogurt **(10g protein)**</li><li>1 cup unsweetened almond milk **(1g protein)**</li><li>1 scoop vanilla protein powder **(20g protein)**</li><li>1 tablespoon chia seeds **(2g protein)**</li><li>1 tablespoon peanut butter **(4g protein)**</li><li>Season to taste</li></ul>	Optional: ½ cup fresh berries or 1 tablespoon sliced almonds. Refrigerator Option: Refrigerate overnight oats in an airtight container or mason jar for up to 4-5 days. Add fresh fruit or nuts/granola just before serving. Freeze Option: Freeze individual portions in a freezer safe container for up to 2 months. Thaw in the fridge, stir before serving.

DIRECTIONS

1. Combine the Ingredients:
   In a mason jar or bowl, add the oats, Greek yogurt, almond milk, protein powder, chia seeds, and peanut butter.

2. Mix Thoroughly:
   Stir the mixture until all ingredients are well combined and the protein powder is fully incorporated.

3. Refrigerate Overnight:
   Cover the container and refrigerate for at least 6 hours or overnight to allow the oats to soften and absorb the liquid.

4. Serve and Garnish:
   In the morning, stir the oats and add fresh berries or sliced almonds as optional toppings.

CHICKEN AND EGG BREAKFAST SANDWICH

BUILD A STRONGER YOU! **1** SERVING **36g** PROTEIN

INGREDIENTS	NOTES
<ul><li>3 oz grilled chicken breast **(26g protein)**</li><li>1 large egg **(6g protein)**</li><li>1 whole-grain English muffin **(4g protein)**</li><li>1 tsp olive oil or butter (for cooking the egg)</li></ul>	Optional: 1 slice of cheese **(5g protein)**, avocado slices, or hot sauce for added flavor. Refrigerator Option: Wrap in saran wrap or foil and refrigerate for 1-2 days. Heat in an oven for best quality.

DIRECTIONS

1. Prepare the Chicken:
• If using pre-cooked grilled chicken, heat it in a skillet or microwave until warm.
• If cooking fresh chicken, season it with salt and pepper (or your favorite spices) and grill it on medium heat for about 5-7 minutes per side, until fully cooked.

2. Toast the Muffin:
  Split the English muffin and toast it in a toaster or on a skillet until golden brown.

3. Cook the Egg:
• Heat olive oil or butter in a small non-stick skillet over medium heat.
• Crack the egg into the skillet and fry it for 2-3 minutes for a sunny-side-up egg, or flip it for a firmer yolk.

4. Assemble the Sandwich:
• Place the bottom half of the English muffin on a plate.
• Layer with the grilled chicken breast.
• Add the fried egg on top of the chicken.
• (**Optional**) Place a slice of cheese or avocado slices on the egg.
• Cover with the top half of the English muffin.

STEAK AND EGGS
BREAKFAST

HEALTH IS WEALTH!	**1** SERVING	**39g** PROTEIN

INGREDIENTS	NOTES
• 4 oz grilled steak **(26g protein)** • 2 large eggs **(12g protein)** • 1/4 cup sautéed mushrooms **(1g protein)**	Optional: Salt, pepper, olive oil (for cooking). Refrigerator Option: Store in an airtight container for 1-2 days. Freeze Option: Freeze steak & eggs separately for up to 1 month.

DIRECTIONS

1. Cook the Steak:
• Season the steak with salt and pepper.
• Heat a grill or grill pan over medium-high heat.
• Cook the steak to your desired doneness, about 4-5 minutes per side for medium-rare, or longer for more well-done steak.
• Remove the steak from the grill and let it rest for 5 minutes before slicing it.

2. Sauté the Mushrooms:
• While the steak is resting, heat a small pan over medium heat and add a drizzle of olive oil (if desired).
• Add the mushrooms and sauté them for 3-4 minutes, stirring occasionally, until softened and slightly browned.
• Season with a pinch of salt and pepper.

3. Cook the Eggs:
• In a separate pan, heat a small amount of olive oil or butter over medium heat.
• Crack the eggs into the pan and fry them to your preferred style (sunny-side-up, over-easy, or scrambled). Season with salt and pepper to taste.

4. Assemble the Plate:
  Arrange the cooked steak on a plate, place the fried eggs next to the steak, top with sautéed mushrooms.

HIGH-PROTEIN BAGEL SANDWICH

<table>
<tr><td>FOCUS ON GROWTH!</td><td>1
SERVING</td><td>31g
PROTEIN</td></tr>
</table>

INGREDIENTS	NOTES
• 1 whole-grain bagel **(10g protein)** • 2 oz smoked salmon **(13g protein)** (Note: Smoked salmon is ready-to-eat and not raw) • 1 large egg **(6g protein)** • 1 tbsp cream cheese **(2g protein)**	Optional: Fresh dill or capers for garnish. Refrigerator Option: Store for 1-2 days. Reheat the egg and bagel, and assemble when ready to serve. Do not freeze.

DIRECTIONS

1. Toast the Bagel:
  Slice the whole-grain bagel in half and toast it until golden and slightly crispy.

2. Cook the Egg:
• Heat a small amount of oil or butter in a pan over medium heat.
• Crack the egg into the pan and fry it until the white is set but the yolk is still runny (or cook it to your desired doneness).

3. Assemble the Sandwich:
• Spread cream cheese on both of the toasted bagel halves.
• Layer the smoked salmon on one half of the bagel.
• Place the cooked egg on top of the salmon.

4. Finish the Sandwich:
  Top with the other half of the bagel. Optionally, garnish with fresh dill or capers for added flavor.

5. Serve and Enjoy:
  Serve immediately and enjoy this high-protein, savory breakfast sandwich!

TACO BREAKFAST BOWL

1
SERVING

37g
PROTEIN

INGREDIENTS	NOTES
<ul><li>2 large eggs **(12g protein)**</li><li>2 oz lean ground turkey or beef **(20g protein)**</li><li>1/4 cup black beans **(3.5g protein)**</li><li>1/4 cup diced tomatoes **(0.5g protein)**</li><li>1 tbsp salsa</li><li>1/4 avocado **(1g protein)**</li><li>1 tsp taco seasoning</li><li>Season to taste</li></ul>	Refrigerator Option: Store for 2-3 days. Freeze Option: Store in an airtight container for up to 1 month.

DIRECTIONS

1. Cook the Ground Turkey or Beef:
• In a pan over medium heat, cook the lean ground turkey or beef, breaking it up into small pieces as it cooks.
• Once cooked through (about 5-7 minutes), add the taco seasoning and a splash of water to help it coat the meat evenly. Stir to combine.
2. Scramble the Eggs:
• In a separate pan, heat a small amount of oil over medium heat.
• Crack the eggs into the pan, and scramble until fully cooked (about 2-3 minutes). Season with a pinch of salt and pepper.
3. Assemble the Taco Bowl:
• In a bowl, add the scrambled eggs, seasoned ground turkey or beef, and black beans.
• Top with diced tomatoes, salsa, and avocado.
4. Serve and Enjoy:
  Mix everything together, or keep the layers separate for a fun presentation!

LUNCH

Lunch is key to maintaining energy, focus, and balanced blood sugar throughout the day. A nutritious midday meal prevents fatigue, supports mental clarity, and curbs overeating later. Choosing wholesome, nutrient-dense foods helps sustain energy and keeps you performing at your best.

COTTAGE CHEESE AND TURKEY WRAPS

INGREDIENTS	NOTES
• ½ cup low-fat cottage cheese **(14g protein)** • 3 slices deli turkey **(15g protein)** • 1 large lettuce leaf or 1 low-carb tortilla (optional) **(1g protein)** • Optional: 1 tsp Dijon mustard	Refrigerator Option: Store in an airtight container for up to 1-2 days. Freeze Option: Not recommended, as wraps tend to get soggy after freezing.

DIRECTIONS

1. Lay Out the Turkey Slices:
  Place the turkey slices flat on a clean cutting board or plate.

2. Add the Cottage Cheese:
• Spoon the cottage cheese onto each turkey slice and spread evenly.
• If using Dijon mustard, spread it over the turkey first before adding the cottage cheese for extra flavor.

3. Roll the Wraps:
• Starting at one end, roll each turkey slice tightly to form a wrap.
• If you prefer a bigger wrap, use a lettuce leaf or low-carb tortilla to hold the turkey and cottage cheese.

4. Serve and Enjoy:
  Place the wraps on a plate and serve immediately, or store in an airtight container in the refrigerator for up to 1-2 days.

SALMON AND VEGGIE POWER BOWL

INGREDIENTS	NOTES
• 4 oz salmon fillet, cooked **(28g protein)** • 1 cup steamed broccoli **(3g protein)** • ½ cup cooked quinoa **(4g protein)** • ¼ avocado, sliced **(1g protein)** • 2 tbsp olive oil (optional: drizzle for flavor) • Salt, pepper, and lemon juice to taste	Refrigerator Option: Store the salmon, quinoa, and vegetables in an airtight container for up to 3 days. Freeze Option: Freeze the salmon and quinoa separately for up to 3 months. Reheat in the oven or microwave, then assemble the bowl when ready to serve.

DIRECTIONS

1. Cook the Salmon:
 Season the salmon with salt and pepper. Pan-sear, bake, or grill for 8-10 minutes, or until cooked through and flaky.

2. Prepare the Veggies and Quinoa:
 Steam the broccoli and cook the quinoa according to package instructions.

3. Assemble the Power Bowl:
 In a bowl, layer the cooked quinoa, steamed broccoli, and avocado slices. Place the cooked salmon on top.

4. Add Flavor and Serve:
 Drizzle with olive oil, sprinkle with lemon juice, and serve immediately for a hearty, high-protein meal.

GRILLED CHICKEN & AVOCADO SANDWICH

STAY MOTIVATED!

1 SERVING

46g PROTEIN

INGREDIENTS	NOTES
<ul><li>4 oz grilled chicken breast **(33g protein)**</li><li>2 slices whole-grain bread **(6g protein)**</li><li>2 slices of tomato</li><li>2 tbsp mashed avocado **(1g protein)**</li><li>1 slice reduced-fat Swiss cheese **(6g protein)**</li><li>1 handful of spinach or arugula</li><li>1 tsp Dijon mustard</li><li>Season to taste</li></ul>	Refrigerator Option: Store in an airtight container for up to 1 day. Keep the sandwich components separate if possible to avoid sogginess. Freeze Option: Not recommended, as the sandwich components will not maintain their texture when frozen.

DIRECTIONS

1. Assemble the Sandwich:
• Spread the mashed avocado on one slice of the bread.
• Layer the grilled chicken, cheddar cheese, tomato slices, and optional greens on top.

2. Toast the Sandwich:
 Top with the second slice of bread. If desired, grill the sandwich in a pan or sandwich press for 2-3 minutes per side until the bread is golden and the cheese is melted.

3. Serve and Enjoy:
 Cut the sandwich in half and serve warm or at room temperature.

CHICKEN AND BLACK BEAN NACHOS

DON'T STOP YET!

1
SERVING

44g
PROTEIN

INGREDIENTS	NOTES
• 4 oz grilled chicken breast, diced **(26g protein)** • ½ cup black beans, rinsed and drained **(7g protein)** • 1 oz shredded cheddar or Mexican blend cheese **(7g protein)** • 8 baked tortilla chips **(2g protein)** • 2 tbsp Greek yogurt **(2g protein)** • 2 tbsp salsa	Optional Toppings: Diced jalapeños, green onions, or cilantro Refrigerator Option: Store in an airtight container for up to 2 days. Freeze Option: Not recommended.

DIRECTIONS

1. Assemble the Nachos:
• Preheat your oven to 375°F. Arrange the tortilla chips on an oven-safe plate or small baking sheet.
• Evenly distribute the diced chicken, black beans, and shredded cheese over the chips.

2. Bake the Nachos:
  Place the nachos in the oven and bake for 5-7 minutes, or until the cheese is fully melted.

3. Add Toppings:
  Remove from the oven and top with Greek yogurt, salsa, and any optional toppings like jalapeños or green onions.

4. Serve Immediately:
  Enjoy as a high-protein snack or light meal.

TUNA AND CHICKPEA SALAD

YOU WERE BUILT FOR THIS!

1
SERVING

49
PROTEIN

INGREDIENTS	NOTES
<ul><li>1 can tuna in water, drained **(25g protein)**</li><li>1 cup chickpeas **(24g protein)**</li><li>2 cups arugula</li><li>½ cucumber, diced</li><li>¼ red onion, thinly sliced</li><li>2 tbsp olive oil</li><li>Juice of 1 lemon</li><li>Season to taste</li></ul>	Refrigerator Option: Store in an airtight container for up to 2 days. Freeze Option: Not recommended, as the texture of the tuna and chickpeas will change when frozen.

DIRECTIONS

1. Prepare the Salad Base:
 In a large bowl, combine the tuna, chickpeas, arugula, cucumber, and red onion.

2. Dress the Salad:
 Drizzle the olive oil and lemon juice over the salad ingredients. Toss everything together until well combined.

3. Serve and Enjoy:
 Serve the salad immediately as a light and protein-packed meal.

DINNER

Dinner is key for restoring energy, aiding muscle recovery, and balancing blood sugar. It provides an opportunity to nourish your body with essential nutrients, promotes better sleep, and helps prevent late-night snacking.

GRILLED CHICKEN AND QUINOA SALAD

NO PAIN, NO GAIN!

1 SERVING

65g PROTEIN

INGREDIENTS	NOTES
<ul><li>1 large chicken breast (6 oz) **(52g protein)**</li><li>1 cup cooked quinoa **(8g protein)**</li><li>2 cups spinach **(2g protein)**</li><li>½ cup cherry tomatoes, halved **(1g protein)**</li><li>½ cucumber, diced</li><li>2 tbsp feta cheese **(2g protein)**</li><li>2 tbsp olive oil</li><li>Juice of 1 lemon</li><li>Salt and pepper to taste</li></ul>	Refrigerator Option: Store in an airtight container for up to 3-4 days. Freeze Option: Not recommended for the salad portion, but you can freeze grilled chicken and quinoa separately for up to 3 months. Thaw and reassemble when ready to serve.

DIRECTIONS

1. Cook the Chicken:
• Preheat a grill or skillet over medium heat. Season the chicken breast with salt, pepper, and any preferred herbs or spices.
• Grill or cook the chicken for 5-7 minutes per side, or until the internal temperature reaches 165°F (75°C). Set aside to rest for 5 minutes before dicing.

2. Cook the Quinoa:
• Rinse the quinoa thoroughly under cold water to remove any bitterness.
• In a small pot, combine ½ cup quinoa with 1 cup water. Bring to a boil, reduce to a simmer, and cover. Cook for 15 minutes or until the water is absorbed. Fluff with a fork and let cool.

3. Prepare the Salad:
• In a large bowl, add the spinach, cherry tomatoes, cucumber, and cooked quinoa.
• Top the salad with diced chicken and sprinkle with feta cheese. Drizzle olive oil and lemon juice over the top. Toss gently to combine.

TURKEY AND BLACK BEAN CHILI

INGREDIENTS	NOTES
<ul><li>1 lb ground turkey **(22g protein)** per serving</li><li>1 can black beans, rinsed **(14g protein)**</li><li>1 can kidney beans, rinsed **(13g protein)**</li><li>1 can diced tomatoes (14 oz) **(1g protein)**</li><li>1 onion, diced **(1g protein)**</li><li>1 bell pepper, diced **(1g protein)**</li><li>2 tbsp chili powder</li><li>1 tsp cumin</li><li>1 cup chicken broth **(2g protein)**</li></ul>	Optional Toppings: Greek yogurt **(10g protein)** per ½ cup) Avocado **(1g protein)** per 2 tbsp) Refrigerator Option: Store in an airtight container for up to 4-5 days. Freeze Option: Freeze in an airtight container or freezer bag for up to 3 months. Thaw overnight in the fridge and reheat thoroughly.

DIRECTIONS

1. Sauté the Vegetables:
Heat a small pot over medium heat and add a drizzle of oil. Add the diced onion and bell pepper. Cook for 3-4 minutes until softened and fragrant.

2. Cook the Turkey:
Add the ground turkey to the pot and break it up with a spoon. Cook for 5-7 minutes until browned and fully cooked.

3. Add the Chili Base:
Stir in the chili powder, cumin, diced tomatoes, black beans, kidney beans, and chicken broth.

4. Simmer:
Reduce the heat to low, cover the pot, and simmer the chili for 20-30 minutes, stirring occasionally to prevent sticking.

5. Serve and Enjoy:
Taste and adjust seasoning if needed. Serve hot with optional toppings like Greek yogurt or avocado.

SALMON WITH LENTILS AND STEAMED BROCCOLI

MAKE IT HAPPEN!	**1** SERVING	**55g** PROTEIN

INGREDIENTS	NOTES
• 1 salmon fillet (6 oz) **(34g protein)** • 1 cup cooked lentils **(18g protein)** • 1 cup steamed broccoli **(3g protein)** • 1 tbsp olive oil • Juice of 1 lemon • 1 tsp garlic powder • 1 tsp smoked paprika	Refrigerator Option: Store in an airtight container for up to 2-3 days. Freeze Option: Not recommended for the cooked broccoli, but you can freeze salmon and lentils separately for up to 2-3 months. Reheat the salmon gently in the oven or on the stove.

DIRECTIONS

1. Prepare the Salmon:
• Preheat the oven to 375°F (190°C).
• Season the salmon fillet with garlic powder, smoked paprika, salt, and pepper on both sides.
• Place the salmon on a baking sheet lined with parchment paper or foil.

2. Bake the Salmon:
Bake the salmon in the preheated oven for 12-15 minutes, or until it is cooked through and flakes easily with a fork.

3. Prepare the Lentils:
• While the salmon is baking, heat the cooked lentils in a small saucepan over medium heat. Stir occasionally until heated through.
• Drizzle with a bit of olive oil for added flavor.

4. Steam the Broccoli:
Steam the broccoli until tender, about 4-5 minutes. You can do this using a steamer basket over boiling water or in the microwave.

5. Assemble the Plate:
Once everything is cooked, place the lentils on the plate and arrange the steamed broccoli and salmon next to them. Drizzle olive oil and lemon juice over the broccoli and lentils.

6. Serve and Enjoy!

SHRIMP STIR-FRY WITH EDAMAME

<table>
<tr><td>BE PROUD OF YOURSELF!</td><td>1
SERVING</td><td>57g
PROTEIN</td></tr>
</table>

INGREDIENTS	NOTES
<ul><li>6 oz shrimp, peeled and deveined **(36g protein)**</li><li>1 cup edamame, shelled **(17g protein)**</li><li>2 cups mixed stir-fry veggies (bell peppers, snap peas, carrots) **(2g protein)**</li><li>2 tbsp soy sauce **(2g protein)**</li><li>1 tbsp sesame oil</li><li>1 tsp minced garlic</li></ul>	Refrigerator Option: Store in an airtight container for up to 2 days. Freeze Option: Not recommended for the stir-fry with edamame, as shrimp can lose texture after freezing. However, you can freeze the cooked shrimp separately for up to 2-3 months.

DIRECTIONS

1. Prepare the Shrimp:
• Heat a large wok or skillet over medium-high heat and add sesame oil.
• Once hot, add the minced garlic and sauté for 30 seconds until fragrant.

2. Cook the Shrimp:
Add the shrimp to the pan and cook for 3-4 minutes until pink and cooked through. Remove them from the pan and set aside.

3. Stir-Fry the Vegetables:
In the same pan, add the mixed stir-fry vegetables and cook for 3-4 minutes, stirring occasionally, until the vegetables are tender-crisp.

4. Add the Edamame and Soy Sauce:
Stir in the shelled edamame and soy sauce. Cook for an additional 2-3 minutes until the edamame is heated through.

5. Combine and Serve:
• Return the cooked shrimp to the pan and toss everything together until well mixed and heated through.
• Serve immediately, either on its own or over rice if desired.

BEEF AND VEGGIE
STUFFED BELL PEPPERS

YOU'RE RESILIENT! | **1** SERVING | **40g** PROTEIN

INGREDIENTS	NOTES
<ul><li>4 large bell peppers **(2g protein)** per pepper</li><li>1 lb lean ground beef **(22g protein)** per serving</li><li>1 cup cooked quinoa **(8g protein)**</li><li>1 can diced tomatoes (14 oz) **(1g protein)**</li><li>1 cup spinach, chopped **(1g protein)**</li><li>½ cup mozzarella cheese **(6g protein)**</li></ul>	Refrigerator Option: Store in an airtight container for up to 3-4 days. Freeze Option: Freeze stuffed bell peppers individually in a single layer on a baking sheet, then transfer to a freezer bag for up to 3 months. Reheat in the oven at 375°F for 25-30 minutes or until heated through.

DIRECTIONS

1. Preheat the Oven:
Preheat the oven to 375°F (190°C).

2. Prepare the Bell Peppers:
Slice the tops off the bell peppers and remove the seeds. Set aside.

3. Cook the Ground Beef:
In a skillet over medium heat, cook the ground beef until browned, breaking it up as it cooks. Drain any excess fat.

4. Prepare the Stuffing:
In a bowl, combine the cooked ground beef, cooked quinoa, diced tomatoes, and chopped spinach. Stir until everything is well mixed.

5. Stuff the Peppers:
• Stuff each bell pepper with the beef and quinoa mixture, pressing down gently to pack it in.
• Place the stuffed peppers in a baking dish and top with mozzarella cheese.

6. Bake:
Bake the stuffed peppers in the preheated oven for 25-30 minutes, or until the peppers are tender and the cheese is melted and bubbly.

7. Serve and Enjoy:
Serve the stuffed peppers hot and enjoy this hearty, protein-packed meal!

GREEK YOGURT CHICKEN CURRY

EMBRACE THE CHALLENGE!

1
SERVING

55g
PROTEIN

INGREDIENTS	NOTES
<ul><li>4oz chicken breast, diced **(33g protein)**</li><li>1 cup plain Greek yogurt **(20g protein)**</li><li>1 tbsp curry powder</li><li>1 tsp minced garlic</li><li>1 tsp minced ginger</li><li>2 cups spinach **(2g protein)**</li></ul>	Optional: brown rice **(5g protein)** Refrigerator Option: Store in an airtight container for up to 3 days. Freeze Option: Freeze the chicken curry in an airtight container for up to 2-3 months. Thaw in the fridge overnight and reheat on the stove, adding a little water or broth if needed to loosen it.

DIRECTIONS

1. Cook the Chicken:
• In a large skillet, heat a small amount of oil over medium heat.
• Add the minced garlic and ginger and cook for 1-2 minutes until fragrant.
• Add the diced chicken and cook for 5-7 minutes until browned and cooked through.

2. Add the Curry Flavor:
• Stir in the curry powder and cook for another minute to toast the spices.
• Add the Greek yogurt and stir until well combined, creating a creamy curry sauce.

3. Add the Spinach:
Stir in the spinach and cook for 2-3 minutes until it wilts and is incorporated into the curry sauce.

4. Serve:
Serve the curry hot over the diced chicken, optionally over brown rice or with naan for extra flavor and texture.

BAKED TOFU WITH SESAME NOODLES

<table>
<tr><td>**BELIEVE IN YOU!**</td><td>**1**
SERVING</td><td>**48g**
PROTEIN</td></tr>
</table>

INGREDIENTS	NOTES
• 1 block firm tofu, cubed **(36g protein)** • 8 oz whole-wheat noodles **(12g protein)** • 1 tbsp sesame oil • 2 tbsp soy sauce • 2 cups stir-fry veggies	Refrigerator Option: Store in an airtight container for up to 3 days. Freeze Option: Not recommended for the noodles, but you can freeze the tofu separately for up to 2 months. Reheat by pan-frying for best texture.

DIRECTIONS

1. Prepare the Tofu:
• Preheat the oven to 400°F (200°C).
• Cube the tofu and place it on a baking sheet lined with parchment paper. Drizzle with soy sauce and bake for 20 minutes, flipping halfway through.

2. Cook the Noodles:
  Cook the whole-wheat noodles according to package instructions. Drain and set aside.

3. Stir-Fry the Veggies:
  In a large skillet, heat the sesame oil over medium-high heat. Add the stir-fry veggies and cook for 3-4 minutes until tender-crisp.

4. Combine the Noodles and Tofu:
  Add the cooked noodles and baked tofu to the skillet. Stir everything together and drizzle with additional soy sauce to taste.

5. Serve and Enjoy:
  Serve the stir-fry immediately, topped with a sprinkle of sesame seeds if desired.

GROUND TURKEY AND SPINACH QUESADILLA

PROGRESS TAKES PATIENCE!

1
SERVING

53g
PROTEIN

INGREDIENTS	NOTES
<ul><li>2 large whole-wheat tortillas **(8g protein)**</li><li>5 oz lean ground turkey **(30g protein)**</li><li>1 cup fresh spinach **(1g protein)**</li><li>½ cup shredded mozzarella cheese **(14g protein)**</li><li>1 tsp garlic powder</li><li>1 tsp olive oil</li><li>Optional: avocado slices for garnish **(1g protein)**</li></ul>	Refrigerator Option: Store in an airtight container or wrap tightly in foil for up to 3 days. Freeze Option: Slice the quesadilla into portions. Place pieces in a single layer on a baking sheet and freeze for 1-2 hours. Once frozen, transfer slices to a freezer-safe bag or airtight container. Store for up to 2 months.

DIRECTIONS

1. Cook the Turkey and Spinach:
• Heat olive oil in a skillet over medium heat.
• Add the ground turkey and cook, breaking it apart with a spatula, until fully browned (5-7 minutes).
• Stir in the garlic powder and spinach, cooking until the spinach is wilted (1-2 minutes).
2. Assemble the Quesadilla:
• Place one tortilla in a clean, dry skillet over medium heat.
• Sprinkle half of the shredded mozzarella cheese evenly over the tortilla.
• Spread the cooked turkey and spinach mixture over the cheese.
• Top with the remaining cheese and place the second tortilla on top.
3. Cook the Quesadilla:
 Cook for 2-3 minutes per side, pressing down gently with a spatula, until the tortillas are golden brown and crispy.
4. Serve and Enjoy:
 Transfer to a cutting board, slice into wedges, and serve warm with optional avocado slices.

PORK TENDERLOIN W/ SWEET POTATO MASH & GREEN BEANS

REMEMBER YOUR GOALS!

1 SERVING

48g PROTEIN

INGREDIENTS	NOTES
<ul><li>1 pork tenderloin (6 oz per serving) **(44g protein)**</li><li>1 large sweet potato **(2g protein)**</li><li>1 cup green beans **(2g protein)**</li><li>1 tbsp honey</li><li>1 tbsp Dijon mustard</li></ul>	Refrigerator Option: Store in an airtight container for up to 3-4 days. Freeze Option: Freeze pork tenderloin and sweet potato mash separately for up to 3 months. Reheat the pork in the oven at 350°F and the mashed sweet potatoes in the microwave or stovetop.

DIRECTIONS

1. Cook the Pork Tenderloin:
• Preheat the oven to 400°F (200°C). Season the pork tenderloin with salt and pepper.
• Roast the pork for 20-25 minutes, or until it reaches an internal temperature of 145°F (63°C).

2. Prepare the Sweet Potato Mash:
• While the pork cooks, peel and chop the sweet potato. Boil it in salted water for 10-15 minutes, or until fork-tender.
• Mash the sweet potato with a fork or potato masher. Season with salt and pepper to taste.

3. Steam the Green Beans:
  Steam the green beans until tender, about 4-5 minutes.

4. Prepare the Glaze:
  In a small bowl, mix the honey and Dijon mustard together to create a glaze.

5. Serve and Enjoy:
  Serve the roasted pork tenderloin with the mashed sweet potatoes and green beans, drizzling the honey mustard glaze over the pork.

COTTAGE CHEESE AND SPINACH STUFFED CHICKEN

<table>
<tr><td>BUILD A STRONGER YOU!</td><td>1
SERVING</td><td>41g
PROTEIN</td></tr>
</table>

INGREDIENTS	NOTES
• 4 oz chicken breast **(33g protein)** • ¼ cup cottage cheese **(7g protein)** • ½ cup chopped spinach **(1g protein)** • ½ tsp garlic powder • ½ tsp dried oregano	Refrigerator Option: Store in an airtight container for up to 3-4 days. Freeze Option: Freeze the cooked chicken (without the stuffing) for up to 3 months. Reheat in the oven at 375°F, covering with foil to prevent drying out.

DIRECTIONS

1. Preheat the Oven:
 Preheat your oven to 375°F (190°C).

2. Prepare the Spinach and Cottage Cheese Filling:
 In a small bowl, mix together the cottage cheese, chopped spinach, garlic powder, and oregano. Season with salt and pepper to taste.

3. Prepare the Chicken:
 Using a sharp knife, carefully slice a pocket into the center of each chicken breast, being sure not to cut all the way through.

4. Stuff the Chicken:
 Stuff each chicken breast with the cottage cheese and spinach mixture, pressing gently to secure the filling inside.

5. Sear the Chicken:
• Heat the olive oil in a large oven-safe skillet over medium-high heat.
• Once hot, add the stuffed chicken breasts and sear for 2-3 minutes on each side until golden brown.

6. Bake the Chicken:
 Transfer the skillet to the preheated oven and bake for 20-25 minutes, or until the chicken is fully cooked (internal temperature of 165°F/74°C).

7. Serve and Enjoy:
• Remove the chicken from the oven and let it rest for 5 minutes before slicing.
• Serve the stuffed chicken with your favorite side dishes and enjoy!

SNACKS

High-protein snacks support workouts by providing steady energy, aiding muscle repair, and promoting muscle growth. They help prevent energy crashes and support recovery post-workout by rebuilding muscle tissue. These snacks also improve focus, reduce fatigue, and help maintain lean muscle mass.

TUNA SALAD AND CRACKERS

RESULTS REQUIRE EFFORT!	**1** SERVING	**30g** PROTEIN

INGREDIENTS	NOTES
<ul><li>1 can tuna in water, drained **(26g protein)**</li><li>1 tbsp light mayonnaise</li><li>1 tbsp plain Greek yogurt **(2g protein)**</li><li>1 tsp Dijon mustard</li><li>½ cup diced celery or pickles **(1g protein)**</li><li>5 whole-grain crackers **(6g protein)**</li></ul>	Refrigerator Option: Store the tuna salad in an airtight container for up to 2 days. Store the crackers separately to prevent them from becoming soggy. Freeze Option: Not recommended, as the tuna salad may become watery upon thawing.

DIRECTIONS

1. Prepare the Tuna Mixture:
• In a medium-sized bowl, add the drained tuna.
• Stir in mayonnaise, Greek yogurt, Dijon mustard, and diced celery or pickles until well combined.

2. Arrange the Crackers:
  Place the whole-grain crackers on a serving plate.

3. Assemble the Tuna Salad and Crackers:
  Either spoon the tuna salad onto each cracker or serve the salad in a small bowl alongside the crackers for dipping.

4. Serve and Enjoy:
  Serve immediately for a fresh, protein-packed snack or meal. Refrigerate leftovers for up to 2 days.

HARD BOILED EGGS
WITH CHEESE

1
SERVING

32g
PROTEIN

INGREDIENTS	NOTES
• 3 large eggs **(18g protein)** • 1 oz cheddar cheese, cubed or sliced **(7g protein)** • 1 oz low-fat string cheese **(7g protein)**	Refrigerator Option: Store the boiled eggs in the refrigerator for up to one week. Keep eggs in their shells for freshness. Freeze Option: Not recommended, as the texture of the egg whites changes when frozen.

DIRECTIONS

1. Boil the Eggs:
• Place the eggs in a saucepan and cover with water.
• Bring the water to a boil, then reduce to a simmer and cook for 9-12 minutes, depending on how firm you prefer the yolks.
• Once cooked, drain the water and transfer the eggs to a bowl of ice water to cool for 5 minutes.

2. Peel the Eggs:
  Gently tap each egg on a hard surface to crack the shell, then peel it off under running water.

3. Serve with Cheese:
  Slice the eggs in half or quarters and arrange them on a plate with the cheddar cheese cubes and string cheese.

4. Enjoy Immediately!

CHICKEN BREAST FRIES

DEDICATION DRIVES SUCCESS! | **1** SERVING | **48g** PROTEIN

INGREDIENTS	NOTES
• 6 oz chicken breast, cut into strips **(48g protein)** • 1 tsp olive oil • 1 tsp garlic powder • ½ tsp smoked paprika • Salt and pepper to taste	Dip Options: Homemade hummus, barbecue sauce, sweet and sour sauce, ranch dressing, or buffalo sauce. Refrigerator Option: Store in an airtight container for up to 3-4 days. Freeze Option: Freeze cooked chicken strips in a single layer on a baking sheet, then transfer to a freezer bag for up to 3 months. Reheat in the oven or on the stovetop.

DIRECTIONS

1. Season the Chicken:
  In a bowl, toss the chicken breast strips with olive oil, garlic powder, smoked paprika, salt, and pepper.

2. Cook the Chicken:
• Heat a non-stick skillet over medium heat. Add the chicken strips in a single layer.
• Cook for 4-5 minutes per side, or until the chicken is fully cooked and reaches an internal temperature of 165°F.

3. Serve and Enjoy:
  Serve the chicken strips immediately as a snack or with a dipping sauce of your choice.

EDAMAME SURPRISE

<table>
<tr><td>MAKE IT HAPPEN!</td><td>1
SERVING</td><td>32g
PROTEIN</td></tr>
</table>

INGREDIENTS	NOTES
• 1 cup cooked edamame **(17g protein)** • 1 protein bar with at least **(15g protein)**	Refrigerator Option: Store the edamame in an airtight container for up to 2 days. Keep protein bars in a cool, dry place according to the manufacturer's use by date. Freeze Option: Freeze edamame in a freezer bag for up to 3 months. Protein bars can be frozen for up to 2 months.

DIRECTIONS

1. Cook the Edamame:
  If using frozen edamame, steam or microwave according to the package instructions until heated through. Sprinkle with a pinch of salt if desired.

2. Serve with the Protein Bar:
  Pair the cooked edamame with your favorite protein bar for a quick, high-protein snack.

PB&J WITH A TWIST

<table>
<tr><td>BE YOUR OWN ROLE MODEL!</td><td>1
SERVING</td><td>33g
PROTEIN</td></tr>
</table>

INGREDIENTS	NOTES
<ul><li>2 slices of high-protein bread **(10g protein)** per slice)</li><li>2 tbsp natural peanut butter **(8g protein)**</li><li>2 tbsp high-protein Greek yogurt instead of jelly, **(5-6g protein)**</li><li>1 tbsp chia seed jam (optional, adds fiber and flavor)</li></ul>	Bread Options: Ezekiel or Dave's Killer bread. Refrigerator Option: Store the assembled sandwich in an airtight container or wrap it tightly in plastic wrap. It will stay fresh for 1-2 days. Freeze Option: Freezing is not recommended for this sandwich.

DIRECTIONS

1. Spread the Peanut Butter:
  Evenly spread the peanut butter on one slice of bread.

2. Prepare the Greek Yogurt Spread:
• In a small bowl, mix the Greek yogurt with a bit of honey or a dash of protein powder (optional) for added sweetness.
• Spread the Greek yogurt mixture over the second slice of bread.

3. Add the Chia Seed Jam (Optional):
  If using, spread the chia seed jam over the Greek yogurt layer for a fruity twist.

4. Assemble the Sandwich:
• Place the two slices together, ensuring the fillings are evenly distributed.
• Slice in half and serve immediately.

RENEW YOUR MIND

A Guide to Overcoming Procrastination

Overcoming procrastination with exercise often requires a combination of mindset shifts, practical strategies, and small habit changes. Here are some evidence-based tips to help:

1. **Start Small** – A short 5–10 minute workout reduces resistance and builds momentum.

2. **Focus on Immediate Benefits** – Exercise boosts mood instantly. Think about how great you'll feel afterward.

3. **Schedule It** – Treat workouts like appointments to stay accountable.

4. **Use the "2-Minute Rule"** – Commit to a tiny first step, like putting on workout clothes.

5. **Find What You Enjoy** – Stick with activities that feel fun, not like a chore.

6. **Exercise with Others** – A buddy or group makes it more enjoyable and motivating.

7. **Visualize Success** – Picture yourself completing the workout and feeling accomplished.

8. **Remove Barriers** – Prep your gear in advance to make starting easier.

9. **Set Small Goals** – Aim for specific, short-term targets, like a 20-minute walk.

10. **Reward Yourself** – Pair exercise with a small treat, like a favorite show or snack.

11. **Track Progress** – Logging workouts boosts motivation and shows results.

12. **Shift Your Mindset** – See exercise as a privilege, not a chore—an investment in your health.

These simple changes can help you build a lasting exercise habit.

TOP PRE-WORKOUT FOODS
Fuel for Energy and Performance

1. **Bananas**
• Pre-Workout Benefit: Rich in fast-digesting carbohydrates to provide quick energy. High in potassium, which helps prevent muscle cramps and supports nerve function.
• Timing: Ideal 30–60 minutes before exercise.

2. **Oats**
• Pre-Workout Benefit: Packed with complex carbs for sustained energy release. Oats contain beta-glucan, a soluble fiber that slows digestion and maintains stable blood sugar levels during workouts.
• Timing: Eat 1–2 hours before exercising for best results.

3. **Sweet Potatoes**
• Pre-Workout Benefit: Provide complex carbs for long-lasting energy and high levels of vitamin A, which supports immunity and recovery.
• Timing: Best eaten 1–2 hours before workouts, especially for endurance activities.

4. **Rice Cakes with Nut Butter**
• Pre-Workout Benefit: Rice cakes offer quick-digesting carbs, while nut butter adds a small amount of healthy fat for endurance.
• Timing: A light option 30 minutes before a workout.

5. **Greek Yogurt with Berries**
• Pre-Workout Benefit: Combines protein for muscle preservation with carbs from berries for an energy boost. Contains calcium to support muscle contraction.
• Timing: Eat 1 hour before exercising.

6. **Trail Mix (Nuts and Dried Fruit)**
• Pre-Workout Benefit: Dried fruit provides natural sugars for quick energy, while nuts supply healthy fats for sustained stamina.
• Timing: Consume 30 minutes to 1 hour before working out.

7. **Black Coffee**
• Pre-Workout Benefit: Caffeine enhances focus, energy levels, and fat oxidation. It may delay fatigue during workouts.
• Timing: Drink 30 minutes before exercise.

TOP POST- WORKOUT FOODS
Recovery and Muscle Repair

1. **Eggs**
• Post-Workout Benefit: A high-quality complete protein containing all essential amino acids for muscle repair. Rich in choline, which supports brain function.
• Timing: Eat within 30–60 minutes post-workout.

2. **Chicken Breast**
• Post-Workout Benefit: Lean source of protein to rebuild muscle tissue. High in B vitamins, which help convert food into energy.
• Timing: Best paired with a carb like quinoa or rice for glycogen replenishment.

3. **Quinoa**
• Post-Workout Benefit: A complex carbohydrate that replenishes glycogen stores. Also contains protein for muscle repair and recovery.
• Timing: Ideal when combined with a protein source post-exercise.

4. **Salmon**
• Post-Workout Benefit: Rich in omega-3 fatty acids, which reduces inflammation and support joint health. High in protein for muscle repair.
• Timing: Best eaten within 1–2 hours after exercising.

5. **Sweet Potatoes**
• Post-Workout Benefit: Restore glycogen levels with complex carbs and provide potassium to prevent cramping and fatigue.
• Timing: Pair with another protein source post-workout for optimal recovery.

6. **Cottage Cheese**
• Post-Workout Benefit: Contains casein protein, which is slow-digesting and supports muscle recovery during sleep. Also high in calcium and phosphorus for bone health.
• Timing: Ideal for a post-workout snack or before bed.

Recovery and Muscle Repair

(Continued)

7. **Protein Shakes**
• Post-Workout Benefit: A quick and convenient source of complete protein to kickstart muscle repair. Often combined with carbs for glycogen replenishment.
• Timing: Best consumed within 30 minutes after a workout.

8. **Coconut Water**
• Post-Workout Benefit: Hydrates the body and replenishes lost electrolytes like potassium and magnesium, which prevent muscle cramps.
• Timing: Consume immediately after exercise.

9. **Spinach**
• Post-Workout Benefit: High in antioxidants and iron, supporting oxygen transport to muscles and reducing inflammation.
• Timing: Add to meals or smoothies post-workout.

10. **Tart Cherry Juice**
• Post-Workout Benefit: Contains antioxidants and anti-inflammatory compounds that reduce muscle soreness and speed up recovery.
• Timing: Drink within 1–2 hours after intense exercise.

Thank You for Your Support!

We appreciate you for choosing 30 Over Thirty! To help you stay on track with your nutrition and goals, we've created a FREE Food Diary just for you.

Use it daily to:
- Track your meals and protein intake
- Build healthy habits
- Reflect on your mood and progress

Simply scan the QR code to download your FREE food diary and start journaling your journey today!

This is our way of saying thank you for supporting this book. We can't wait to see you crush your goals!